14 Reasons to Quit Smoking

(one for every minute of the day)

Bill Dodds

Meadowbrook Press
Distributed by Simon & Schuster
New York

Library of Congress Cataloging-in-Publication Data

Dodds, Bill.

   1,440 reasons to quit smoking : (one for every minute of the day) / Bill
Dodds.

     p. cm.

   ISBN 0-88166-381-6 (Meadowbrook) ISBN 0-671-31863-2 (Simon &
Schuster)

   1. Cigarette habit—Prevention. 2. Tobacco habit—Prevention. 3.
Tobacco habit—Treatment. 4. Smoking cessation programs. I. Title: One
thousand four hundred forty reasons to quit smoking. II. Title.

HV5740 .D64 2000
613.85—dc21

                                      00-038668

Managing Editor: Christine Zuchora-Walske
Coordinating Editor: Megan McGinnis
Proofreaders: H.J. Giostra, Laurie Anderson
Production Manager: Paul Woods
Desktop Publishing: Danielle White

Published by Meadowbrook Press, 5451 Smetana Drive, Minnetonka, MN
55343

www.meadowbrookpress.com

BOOK TRADE DISTRIBUTION by Simon & Schuster, a division of Simon
and Schuster, Inc., 1230 Avenue of the Americas, New York, NY 10020

04 03 02 01 00   10 9 8 7 6 5 4 3 2

Printed in the United States of America

Dedication

To anyone trying to quit smoking:
I wish you complete success
and a long, happy, and healthy life.

Acknowledgments

We would like to thank the
individuals who served on
reading panels for this project:

L.A. Chell, Paul Driscoll, H.J. Giostra,
Charles L. Grove, S.E. McGinnis, Rosemary
Schmidt, Denise Tiffany, Timothy Tocher,
Debra Tracy, Marvin Wallace

Beating Tobacco,
One Minute at a Time

The Centers for Disease Control and Prevention suggest anyone trying to stop smoking "take quitting one day at a time, even one minute at a time—whatever you need to succeed."

One minute at a time.

Anyone battling an addiction knows a minute can be what it takes.

Anyone battling an addiction knows that in the grip of a craving, it's hard to remember why you wanted to quit in the first place. It's hard to remember a single reason not to give up.

You want a reason. You need a reason. Right here. Right now.

This book offers 1,440 reasons not to light that next cigarette, one for every minute of the day. I wrote it to help you become what you need to be: an ex-smoker. And if you never light that next cigarette, you are—and will remain—an ex-smoker.

Obviously, the book isn't designed to be read from cover to cover. You can open it to any page and find encouraging reasons not to smoke.

The reasons fall into two categories: good stuff and bad stuff. Smoking leads to bad stuff. Quitting is the way to good stuff. You know that, of course. You're no fool. But when the urge to smoke is overwhelming, you might find it difficult to think about anything except taking one more puff.

These are 1,440 reasons not to take that puff.

As someone who has quit smoking and drinking, I know what you're going through. I know the path to success often seems to be measured not just by days or by hours but— truly—by minutes.

And although this book was written for cigarette smokers, most reasons can apply to users of any tobacco. It can help if you're trying to quit smoking cigars or pipes, or using smokeless tobacco.

Becoming tobacco-free may be the hardest challenge you'll ever face. And once you succeed, you'll have every right to be extremely proud of yourself.

You can do this.

You can do this.

You can do this.

When you stop to smell the roses, you'll actually be able to smell them.

Your lungs have been trying to tell you something ever since that first—*gasp, cough*—drag.

You get enough pollution in your lungs just by living in the city.

The princess won't kiss a frog that smells like an ashtray.

The frog can't be kissed if the princess has a cigarette between her lips.

Smoking has been linked to impotence.

You're getting too old for this nonsense.

Doctor's orders.

You promised your spouse you'd quit.

You don't want to tell people you've started up again.

Those wrinkles around your eyes.

No amount of tar is "low" enough.

Your mama is going to be so pleased with you.

Your papa is going to be so proud of you.

Nicotine is used as an insecticide.

Right now, you're an ex-smoker.

Your grandchildren will want you at their high-school graduations.

With over a year's worth of money spent daily on a pack, you could buy a ticket to Paris or fantastic seats at a professional basketball game.

Every smoker quits eventually—one way or another.

You're not going to care if the flight is nonsmoking.

Your taste buds want to get back to work.

No one ever set the house on fire by dropping a bag of sunflower seeds on the couch.

It's time to quit. You know it's time to quit.

You don't want your kids to smoke.

Kissing.

Smoother skin.

It isn't only the good who die young.

Russian roulette has an inevitable outcome, unless the player quits.

Yellow teeth.

You'll be showing those jerks who say you can't quit.

Your body has already started to heal itself.

Nicotine is a drug.

Only God and the tobacco industry really know what is in cigarettes.

Strokes don't always kill; sometimes they severely disable.

Getting better tables at restaurants.

Going back to square one in the quitting process would be the pits.

You don't want to be a quitter when it comes to quitting.

The urge will pass.

Portable oxygen tanks.

Stinky ashtrays.

You want to smoke, but you choose not to.

Your lungs aren't designed to be smoked from the inside out as if they were some kind of ham.

Mints and gum don't really cover smoker's breath.

Watching two-hour movies straight through.

There are darn few eighty-something smokers and not many in their seventies.

Each pack you buy makes tobacco executives richer.

Heart attacks.

You're on your way to being free at last!

Smokers who "eat right and get lots of exercise" are only kidding themselves.

Tobacco use is responsible for nearly 20 percent of all deaths in the United States.

Your next cold won't be so severe.

More women die of lung cancer than of breast cancer.

An extra twenty to twenty-five years added to your life.

Cancer really hurts.

There are millions of ex-smokers who have "been there/done that," and they want you to wear the T-shirt, too.

You know smoking is not only danger-ous, it's also stupid.

Deep down, you *do* care.

The confusion is temporary. In the long run, you'll think even more clearly than before you quit.

All the anxiety you feel during withdrawal burns calories.

No one ever died from losing a night of sleep.

Your spouse doesn't want to go through life without you.

Your children will miss you.

Cleaner walls.

Less expensive drapery-cleaning bills.

Self-satisfaction.

Dropped lit cigarettes can cause fires.

Your grandchildren look up to you.

You remember dead friends who didn't
quit.

A family history of cancer.

Heart attacks are often *extremely* painful.

You're tired of being a drug addict.

You said you'd quit.

That burn hole in your suede jacket.

Standing outside an air-conditioned building to smoke when it's 101° in the shade.

No more middle-of-the-night runs to the convenience store for a pack.

Climbing stairs easily.

Social pressure to quit.

That last smoke was your last one.

Those atrocious taxes on tobacco products.

Your physical exam is coming up.

You bet this time you would succeed.

You wish you had never started.

Tracheotomies.

Lung tissue that's like leather.

Nobody ever died of cravings.

Tobacco company executives' annual bonuses.

You won't have to get your spouse any other birthday present.

This may be the best Mother's Day gift your mom has ever received.

After this, every challenge will seem easier.

There's no way you're going to go through the hell of quitting again.

When you get through this, you're going to buy yourself something *really* nice.

As the American Lung Association points out, "When you can't breathe, nothing else matters."

A burning cigarette contains more than four thousand substances, including forty known to cause cancer.

Carbon monoxide.

Annually, thousands of nonsmokers die of lung cancer because of secondhand smoke.

Carcinogens.

The Environmental Protection Agency (EPA) categorizes secondhand smoke with radon, asbestos, and benzene.

Infants and young children regularly exposed to secondhand smoke are likely to suffer from lower respiratory tract infections, such as pneumonia and bronchitis.

Asthma.

Kids subjected to secondhand smoke often develop a buildup of fluid in the middle ear, a condition that's the most common reason children need surgery.

The level of tar particles in indoor cigarette smoke often exceeds the national outdoor air quality standards established by the EPA.

Starting at age thirty-five, a female smoker is twelve times more likely than a female nonsmoker to die of lung cancer.

Starting at age thirty-five, a female smoker is ten times more likely than a female nonsmoker to die of emphysema or chronic bronchitis.

Smoking during pregnancy causes serious health problems for the unborn child.

A pregnant woman who smokes passes nicotine to her fetus.

A pregnant woman who smokes prevents as much as 25 percent of oxygen from reaching the placenta.

There's a link between moms who smoke and infants and young kids who suffer from asthma.

Moms who smoke pass nicotine through their breast milk to their nursing babies.

Since the 1920s, the tobacco industry has targeted women by using images of freedom, glamour, thinness, and feminism.

Women don't need to smoke to be free, glamorous, thin, or feminist.

Smokers look old prematurely.

The best time to quit is right now.

Stinky coats.

Most nicotine withdrawal symptoms are completely gone in six months.

Cigarette smoking is the single greatest cause of preventable diseases.

Smoking causes more than one thousand deaths per day in the United States.

Pneumonia.

A pack a day doubles your chances of dying between the ages of fifty and sixty.

Two packs a day triples it.

Only 10 percent of doctors in the United States smoke.

Inhaled tobacco contains chemicals used to cultivate tobacco plants.

More than 80 percent of smokers want to stop.

The American Psychiatric Association has called smoking an "organic mental disorder."

Nicotine constricts blood vessels, which increases blood pressure and stimulates the heart, and raises fat levels in the blood.

Injecting even a drop of liquid nicotine would be deadly.

Cigarette smoke contains hydrogen cyanide.

Chemicals are added to make tobacco burn better and taste different.

Smoking reduces vitamin C absorption.

Radioactive materials are found in cigarette smoke. Polonium is the most common.

Mouth cancer.

Tongue cancer.

Bladder cancer.

Kidney cancer.

Cancer of the pancreas.

Cervical cancer.

Peptic ulcers.

Varicose veins.

Hiatal hernia.

Osteoporosis.

Gum disease.

Senility.

Lungs weren't made to inhale carbon monoxide.

Nicotine raises the level of "bad" choles-terol and lowers the level of "good."

No more hoarseness.

Cancer of the larynx is almost exclusive to smokers.

Angina pectoris—chest pains.

Smoking reduces lung capacity.

Smoking lowers your immunity.

No more leg pains.

Less risk of complications after surgery.

Cerebral aneurysms, the ballooning of
artery walls in the brain, afflict smokers
more than nonsmokers.

Vascular diseases can lead to amputations.

Over time, after it's been irritated,
inflamed, and scarred, lung tissue is
destroyed.

You need your larynx to talk.

Fewer bouts of sinusitis.

Increased endurance.

No more coughing fits in the morning.

Living long enough to celebrate your golden anniversary.

The smell of spring rain.

Your pride.

Running for the bus and catching it.

Your nonsmoking car pool.

Clean fingers.

Less need to dust your furniture.

Cheaper life insurance.

Next year, all this will only be a bad memory.

You can join the "if I can do it, anyone can" crowd.

More money for that cruise.

Cheaper dry-cleaning bills.

That little twerp you can't stand has quit.

"Sin" tax.

Only dragons can blow smoke from their noses safely.

Quitting might shut up those annoying politically correct, tree-hugging, tofu-eating coworkers.

Government subsidies for tobacco farmers.

You can still keep your favorite lighter.

No more beef-jerky tongue.

Smoking really doesn't make you look like a cowboy.

Only you can prevent forest fires.

You want a l—o—n—g retirement.

Your grandkid already mimics you.

Then you were a dumb kid. Now you know better.

It's never too late to quit.

Smoke gets in your eyes.

You spent a fortune on those quit-smoking classes.

You're tired of sneaking butts.

Better to quit now than after the heart attack.

It might be hard to hold a cigarette after you've had a stroke.

Smoking may seem like a longtime companion, but it's never been your friend.

No more gravel voice.

You've wanted to quit for a long time.

Quitting cold turkey works.

Facing your dentist without shame.

Disappointing that self-righteous in-law who predicted you'll be smoking till the day you die.

You said you could quit anytime you wanted, and you said you wanted to quit now.

Taking a deep breath not followed by a cough.

The smell and taste of bacon.

No one ever looked in the casket and said, "Well, at least she died skinny."

Spots on x-rays.

Millions of ex-smokers know *exactly* what you're going through.

You're stronger than you realize.

Your fiftieth birthday.

Your sixtieth birthday.

Your seventieth birthday.

Your eightieth birthday.

Your ninetieth birthday.

Your name and photo on a national TV morning show when you hit a hundred.

You'll get to say, "Well, I used to smoke."

It may help your spouse quit smoking.

You told your folks you quit.

There's not going to be a sudden drop in cigarette prices.

No more running to the smoking car during long train trips.

No more hunting for the longest butt in the ashtray when you're out of cigarettes.

You're not invincible.

There's a reason you don't like to think about what it does to your body.

You'll sleep better . . . eventually.

Ex-smoking friends are praying for you.

This may be the worst of it.

Most people *don't* smoke.

This is the when, where, and how you'll win the battle.

A house that smells fresh and clean.

Spray-on upholstery odor-removers don't completely remove smoky smells.

You want to taste spices again.

After quitting, you'll feel like you can do anything.

That exercise machine gathering dust in the bedroom corner.

No more raw throat.

A new lease on life.

The future always looks brighter when it isn't dimmed by smoke.

Annoyed glances and rude comments from nonsmokers in restaurants.

Your spouse makes you go outside to smoke.

You've put a lot of money into social security, and you'd like to be around to use it.

Tar makes strong roads and weak lungs.

Car fresheners don't make your car smell like a nonsmoker's car.

Money for cigarettes diverted to a retirement account will make a lovely nest egg.

Smoking during pregnancy accounts for roughly 20 to 30 percent of all low-birth-weight babies.

Smoking during pregnancy accounts for up to 14 percent of all preterm deliveries.

Smoking during pregnancy accounts for roughly 10 percent of all infant deaths.

Researchers claim smoking increases the risk of SIDS, sudden infant death syndrome.

You want to have a baby.

You're pregnant.

Your wife is pregnant.

You want to cut down on your formalde-hyde intake.

You're tired of lying about your smoking.

You suspect the tobacco companies just might be targeting kids.

The cigarette companies' "free" stuff comes with a hefty price tag.

You still feel bad you didn't succeed the last time you tried to quit.

When it comes to this, quitters are winners.

The past and the future are out of your control. All you have is right now.

You've talked the talk. Now you want to walk the walk.

It's hard to catch your breath with just one lung.

You said last year you'd quit next year. This *is* next year.

You don't want to hear the doctor gently say, "We need to talk."

This war is won one battle at a time.

You know it was stupid to start. You knows it's stupider not to stop.

You don't have to look cool anymore.

There are healthier ways to keep yourself awake.

People are no longer amused with your cigarette tricks.

Enjoying plays without intermissions.

Staying focused during long meetings with your nonsmoking boss.

You'll have more pep.

That new-car smell will last longer.

No more stupid smoking gizmos given to you as gifts.

You know how much smoke makes your hair, clothes, breath, and house stink.

You're going to discover a lot of food *does* taste the way it did when you were a kid.

You know switching to menthol isn't the solution when your throat is sore.

It's time to kick butt.

This might be your worst moment. It could start to get better from here. But you won't know unless you refuse to light up.

You don't want to sit through another quit-smoking class.

You know you've been ignoring what your body's been telling you.

Your body is your temple.

Quitting is like winning a lottery that pays you hundreds of dollars a year for the rest of your life.

You don't want to pick out your pall-bearers just yet.

Many years from now, this will simply be known as Hell Day.

You don't want to disappoint your loved ones.

You don't want to disappoint yourself.

You *do* want to disappoint tobacco company stockholders.

You *can* do your job without a cigarette.

This is a gift you're giving yourself.

Smoking isn't something you really *want* to do.

Cravings go away. Cancer grows.

You know you've been ignoring scare tactics because they really scare you.

Smoking is most illogical, Captain.

People look up to you.

You can book a nonsmoking room at a fancy hotel.

You want to be done with the patches and the gum.

If you have one cigarette now, you'll *really* want another one fifteen minutes from now.

Smoking is selfish.

It'll be great succeeding at the hardest challenge you've ever faced.

Someone you loved deeply died before his time because he smoked.

Oncologists.

You want a better life.

The least educated among us are the ones most likely to smoke.

The beautiful people in cigarette ads don't have oxygen tubes up their noses.

The only way to stop being a drug addict is to stop taking the drug.

The smell of freshly baked bread.

You want to try line dancing.

There are no smokes in the house, and you said you wouldn't buy any more.

You're way too old to sneak cigarettes.

You don't want to disappoint the folks in your quit-smoking class.

You made a pact with a friend who's trying to quit, and you'll be darned if you'll be the first to break it.

Ashes all over your computer keyboard.

You said you'd get in shape.

You'd rather play full-court basketball than H.O.R.S.E.

Smoking makes you feel like a loser.

You have teenagers.

You've had it up to *here* with your mother's comments about your smoking.

You don't have a secret death wish.

It's time to start a new chapter in your life.

Your friends have quit.

Smoking makes it harder to attract members of the opposite sex.

There was that little medical incident you didn't tell anyone about. The one that scared the hell out of you.

You're tired of huddling outside doorways in the middle of winter to have a smoke.

You wouldn't let your dog smoke.

You're tired of smoking.

Smoking because you're angry won't change the situation.

You want to be in control of your life.

Taking brisk walks.

You're tired of the lies.

Being an ex-smoker will be a joy.

Quitting is like having your death
sentence commuted.

You hate smoking.

You hated being a smoker.

It's hard to hold your head high when
you're coughing.

Each cigarette takes an estimated twelve
minutes off your life.

Breathing is good. Not breathing is bad.

You'd like to feel rested for a change.

No more scheduling smoke-breaks.

You won't regret staying an ex-smoker.

You want to live.

Singing at the top of your lungs.

No more throbbing legs and feet.

No more icy hands and feet.

A brighter smile and a great reason to flash it.

There's no better birthday present for yourself or a loved one.

If it's been twenty minutes since your last cigarette, your blood pressure is dropping to normal.

If it's been twenty minutes since your last cigarette, your pulse rate is dropping to normal.

If it's been twenty minutes since your last cigarette, the body temperature of your hands and feet has increased.

If it's been eight hours since your last cigarette, the carbon monoxide level in your blood has dropped to normal.

If it's been eight hours since your last cigarette, the oxygen level in your blood has increased to normal.

If it's been eight hours since your last cigarette, your ability to smell and taste has increased.

If it's been twenty-four hours since your last cigarette, your chances of having a heart attack have decreased.

If it's been forty-eight hours since your last cigarette, your nerve endings are regrowing.

Two weeks to a month after quitting, your circulation will improve.

Two weeks to a month after quitting, walking will be easier.

Two weeks to a month after quitting, your lung function will increase up to 30 percent.

One to nine months after quitting, you'll endure fewer bouts of coughing, sinus congestion, fatigue, and shortness of breath.

One to nine months after quitting, the cilia in your lungs will regrow, increasing your body's ability to handle mucus, clean the lungs, and reduce infection.

One to nine months after quitting, your body's overall energy will increase.

A year after quitting, your excess risk of coronary heart disease will be half that of a smoker.

Five years after quitting, the lung cancer death rate for ex-smokers—who had smoked an average of a pack a day—will decrease by almost half.

Five years after quitting, ex-smokers' risk of cancer of the mouth, throat, and esophagus will be half that of smokers.

Five years to fifteen years after quitting, ex-smokers' risk of stroke will be reduced to that of nonsmokers.

Ten years after quitting, ex-smokers' pre-cancerous cells will be replaced.

Ten years after quitting, ex-smokers' lung cancer death rate will be equivalent to that of nonsmokers.

Ten years after quitting, ex-smokers' risk of cancer of the bladder, kidney, and pancreas will decrease.

Fifteen years after quitting, ex-smokers' risk of coronary heart disease will be that of nonsmokers.

The average weight gain for quitters is five pounds.

Women who smoke reach menopause one to two years earlier than women who are ex-smokers.

Ex-smokers live longer than smokers.

In the game of life, smoking speeds up the time clock.

You don't want your Book of Life to be a short story.

Yul Brynner died of lung cancer at age sixty-five.

Babe Ruth died of cancer at age fifty-three.

Nat "King" Cole died at age forty-five after having surgery for lung cancer.

Actor Chuck Connors, the "Rifleman," died of lung cancer at age seventy-one.

Gary Cooper died at age sixty of lung cancer.

Sammy Davis Jr. died at age sixty-four of lung cancer.

Actress Colleen Dewhurst died at age sixty-seven of lung cancer.

Walt Disney had lung cancer and died at age sixty-five of acute circulatory collapse following an operation to remove a tumor.

Bandleader Jimmy Dorsey died at age fifty-three of lung cancer.

Actor John Candy died of a heart attack at age forty-three.

Ian Fleming, creator of the James Bond novels, died at age fifty-six of a heart attack.

Errol Flynn died of a heart attack at age fifty.

Dancer/choreographer Bob Fosse, a four-packs-a-day smoker, died of a heart attack at age sixty.

Sigmund Freud died at age eighty-three of cancer of the jaw.

Clark Gable died of a heart attack at age fifty-nine.

Jackie Gleason (age seventy-one) and Audrey Meadows (age seventy) of *The Honeymooners* both died of lung cancer.

Talk-show host Arthur Godfrey died of lung cancer at age seventy-nine.

Actor Michael Landon, a four-packs-a-day smoker, died of cancer of the pancreas and liver at age fifty-four.

Alan Jay Lerner, playwright and lyricist (*My Fair Lady* and *Camelot*), died of lung cancer at age sixty-seven.

Actor Lee Marvin died of a heart attack at age sixty-seven.

Wayne McLaren, a cigarette-ad cowboy, died of lung cancer at age fifty-one.

Television actor Doug McClure died of lung cancer at age fifty-six.

Steve McQueen died at age fifty of lung cancer.

Robert Mitchum died of lung cancer at age seventy-nine.

I've Got a Secret game-show host Garry Moore died of emphysema at age seventy-eight.

Edward R. Murrow died of lung cancer on the day before his fifty-seventh birthday.

Actor/singer Bert Parks died of lung cancer at age seventy-seven.

Actor George Peppard died at age sixty-five of complications arising from cancer treatment.

Actor Vincent Price died of lung cancer at age eighty-two.

Anne Ramsey, actress in the movie *Throw Mama from the Train*, died of throat cancer at age fifty-nine.

Newscaster Harry Reasoner died of lung cancer and pneumonia at age sixty-eight.

Actress Lee Remick died of lung and liver cancer at age fifty-five.

Actor Robert Shaw (*The Sting* and *Jaws*) died of a heart attack at age fifty-one.

The Twilight Zone creator, writer, and host Rod Serling died of heart disease at age fifty-one.

Actor Jack Soo (*Barney Miller*) died of cancer of the esophagus at age sixty-three.

Television host Ed Sullivan died of lung cancer at age seventy-two.

Actress Gene Tierney died of emphysema at age seventy.

Actor Spencer Tracy died of lung congestion and a heart attack at age sixty-six.

Singer Mary Wells ("My Guy") died of cancer of the larynx at age forty-nine.

Radio personality and actor Wolfman Jack died of a heart attack at age fifty-seven.

Dick York (first "Darren" on *Bewitched*) died of emphysema at age sixty-three.

Actor Jim Varney—best known as "Ernest" in the *Ernest Goes to* . . . movies —died of lung cancer at the age of fifty.

You've procrastinated long enough.

You've run out of excuses to smoke.

Your spouse quit.

You don't want to want—or need—
another cigarette.

Recently, you have been smoking a lot
more than you used to.

There are better ways to deal with stress.

Your kids look up to you.

All those new antismoking laws.

Your office is nonsmoking.

You can't remember the last time you
really enjoyed a cigarette.

You can't fool your wife.

Your husband may not say anything, but he knows.

Today is almost over. Then you will have made it through today without smoking.

You've forgotten how chocolate *really* tastes.

They're called "cancer sticks" for a good reason.

You've got the tools to succeed. You just have to use them.

You're sick and tired of feeling sick and tired.

Sometimes your heart sounds really loud.

No ex-smoker has ever said, "I wish I hadn't quit."

The human body is a delicate instrument.

Smoking cigarettes has been compared to sucking on a tailpipe.

You want to keep up with your kids.

You want to try to keep up with your grandkids.

You quit once before, and after succeeding this time, you don't ever want to have to quit again.

Burn spots on your necktie.

Your grown kids are worried about you.

Your grown kids want their kids to have a grandparent.

Other members from that old group who smoked in high school aren't doing too well.

Your friends don't like visiting hospitals.

Your friends don't want to go to another funeral.

When the doctor says, "Take a couple of deep breaths," you don't want to go into a coughing jag.

You don't want to treat yourself as one would treat a lab rat.

You wouldn't let a lab rat inhale the junk you've been putting in your lungs.

No one is happier than an addict off the stuff and over the cravings.

You want your life to be better than it is right now.

The thrill is gone, baby.

You're tired of friends giving you news-paper clippings about the ill effects of smoking.

Your dental hygienist will be so happy.

Regular toothpaste will keep your teeth white.

Blood is supposed to carry oxygen, not nicotine.

The only thing you want to take your breath away is romance.

Smoking is—how to put this?—not attractive.

You're in no hurry to use that burial plot you bought.

Smooches shouldn't taste like ashtrays.

Every cigarette you smoke makes you feel like a fool.

Being a "light" smoker is like drinking watered-down arsenic.

Smokers will be green with envy.

Your kids' clothes won't stink anymore.

Your baby has little pink lungs.

Your kids will do as you do, not as you say.

Wait a minute.

You *can* last another sixty seconds.

A minute from now, you'll be so glad you didn't light up.

An hour from now, you'll be so glad you didn't light up.

A day from now, you'll be so glad you didn't light up.

A week from now, you'll be so glad you didn't light up.

A month from now, you'll be so glad you didn't light up.

A year from now, you'll be so glad you didn't light up.

A decade from now, you'll be so glad
you didn't light up.

A quarter of a century from now, you'll
be so glad you didn't light up.

A half century from now, you'll be so
glad you didn't light up.

For the rest of your life, you'll be so glad
you didn't light up.

If someone forced you to inhale tobacco
smoke, you'd sue the pants off him or
her—and win.

The withdrawal headaches will go away.

Crying during withdrawal never killed anyone.

This is one of the greatest opportunities of your life.

No one looks suave spitting a bit of tobacco from the tip of his or her tongue.

A carton costs . . . Oh my goodness! It costs how much now?

One pack a day is 140 cigarettes per week.

One pack a day is six hundred cigarettes per month.

One pack a day is 7,300 cigarettes per year.

One pack a day is 36,500 cigarettes in five years.

One pack a day is seventy-three thousand cigarettes in ten years.

One pack a day is 109,500 cigarettes in fifteen years.

One pack a day is 146,000 cigarettes in twenty years.

One pack a day is 182,500 cigarettes in twenty-five years.

One pack a day is 219,000 cigarettes in thirty years.

One pack a day is 255,500 cigarettes in thirty-five years.

One pack a day is 292,000 cigarettes in forty years.

One pack a day is 328,500 cigarettes in forty-five years.

One pack a day is 365,000 cigarettes in fifty years.

Of course, smoking two packs a day doubles those figures to 14,600 cigarettes in one year and 730,000—almost three-quarters of a million!—in fifty years.

Once you're done with this withdrawal nonsense, you can get on with your life.

Every ex-smoker knows smoking is an addiction.

The smell of a freshly mowed lawn.

The taste of hot buttered popcorn.

Shutting up that nagging little voice in the back of your mind.

The feeling of defeat when you give in and buy another pack.

You are the Master of Your Own Lungs.

Breathing has become a habit.

You love your heart.

The thought of a surgeon cutting you open to operate on your lungs.

Hand-held voice boxes.

You want to join a volleyball league.

Your tennis game has gone to hell.

You want to take swing-dance lessons.

You have no answer when people ask, "Why do you still smoke?"

Your high-school reunion is coming up.

You're tired of making New Year's resolutions you can't keep.

You're not fifteen anymore.

You're not twenty anymore.

You're not thirty anymore.

You're not forty anymore.

You're not fifty anymore.

You're not sixty anymore.

You may not see fifty or sixty or seventy
if you don't quit.

Sooner or later, the piper has to be paid.

Choose life.

Quitting now is like escaping before the car crashes.

You're tired of vowing you're going to quit.

You can change.

If you had to do it over again, you never would have started smoking.

You're tired of feeling guilty.

Your quit-smoking support group will be so proud of you!

It's better to be stressed-out than to be dying.

There are better ways to take a break.

Many forms of relaxation don't come with a warning from the Surgeon General.

No more burns on furniture.

Allergies.

Tooth loss.

Cataracts.

Hearing loss.

Prostate cancer.

Lymphomas.

Gangrene and limb loss.

Better prognosis for surviving surgery.

Cigarettes are toxic when used as intended.

Nicotine alters the modulation of neuro-
transmitters, hormones, and brain, meta-
bolic, and electrical activity.

Researchers say rats will self-administer
nicotine as much as they will cocaine.

The negative moods associated with
withdrawal won't last.

Tobacco is a mood-altering drug.

Better to be angry and irritable during withdrawal than angry and irritable because you could have quit before it was too late.

Annually, the number of people who die because of their tobacco use roughly equals the number of people killed in over a thousand jumbo jet crashes.

It's estimated cigarettes kill half of long-term smokers.

The number of people dependent on nicotine is higher than for any other drug.

Surveys indicate smokers are more stressed-out than nonsmokers.

Ex-smokers report they feel less stressed-out after they have successfully quit.

Cigarette smoke contains acetic acid.

Cigarette smoke contains acetone.

Cigarette smoke contains aluminum.

Cigarette smoke contains ammonia.

Cigarette smoke contains arsenic.

Cigarette smoke contains benzene.

Cigarette smoke contains butane.

Cigarette smoke contains carbon monoxide.

Cigarette smoke contains carbonyl sulfide.

Cigarette smoke contains lead.

Cigarette smoke contains magnesium.

Cigarette smoke contains mercury.

Cigarette smoke contains methane.

Cigarette smoke contains nickel.

Cigarette smoke contains nitric oxide.

Cigarette smoke contains nitrobenzene.

Cigarette smoke contains nitropropane.

Cigarette smoke contains copper.

Cigarette smoke contains DDT.

Cigarette smoke contains formic acid.

Cigarette smoke contains glycerol.

Cigarette smoke contains hydrogen cyanide.

Cigarette smoke contains hydrogen sulfide.

81

Cigarette smoke contains stearic acid.

Cigarette smoke contains titanium.

Cigarette smoke contains urethane.

Cigarette smoke contains vinyl chloride.

Your coworkers are rooting for you.

You want to prove the cynics wrong.

Your self-esteem will soar.

A big gain through some serious pain.

A life not dominated by tobacco.

A schedule not centered around smoke-breaks.

You want your central nervous system's functions to return to normal.

Finding tar residue in your lungs is like finding balls of tar on a polluted beach.

Your smoking embarrasses you.

Any physical side effects of withdrawal won't last.

Any psychological side effects of withdrawal won't last.

Only you know the particular hell you're going through; only you can make certain you never have to go through it again.

Your brain *really* likes oxygen.

You don't want to relapse.

People, memories, places, and situations that spark a craving for tobacco are appropriately called *triggers*.

No more responding to triggers as if you were one of Pavlov's dogs.

It might not seem possible now, but your cravings will decrease over time.

This can be the first step—a huge one—
toward changing your life.

A craving is like an ocean wave: It will
build, crest, break, and diminish.

You don't want to smoke. The urge is
just a reflex.

No more ashes in the carpet.

No more burn holes in the carpet.

No more overflowing ashtrays in the car.

No more bad-tasting breath spray to try
to cover smoker's breath.

No more butts floating in coffee dregs at the bottoms of mugs.

No more searching for excuses about why you haven't quit.

No more rationalizing about when you're going to quit.

No more fearing that your smoking will mean your kids lose a parent too early.

No more friends thinking you're dumb to keep smoking.

No more worrying about getting caught smoking.

No more hunting for matches.

No more muting antismoking ads on TV.

No more fearing news reports on smoking and health.

No more lying about the number of cigarettes you smoke in a day.

No more worrying about how the number of cigarettes you smoke in a day has increased over the years.

No more searching fruitlessly for the perfect cigarette with "low nicotine and great flavor."

No more sucking "low tar, low nicotine" cigarettes down to the filter to get every last bit of tar and nicotine.

No more games of "I'll only smoke when . . ." ("I'm out"; "I'm home"; "I'm bowling"; "I'm at the tavern.")

No more blaming your habit on friends who still smoke.

No more avoidance by friends who don't smoke.

No more offering cockamamie reasons for smoking and acting as if you believe them.

No more tar-coated computer, TV, or VCR parts.

No more rearview mirror coated with a nasty brown film.

No more searching for the smoking areas in airports, train stations, or hospitals.

No more rushing through a meal with nonsmoking friends so you can get out and have a cigarette.

No more standing out in the rain trying to light a cigarette.

No more agreeing when someone comments, "Doesn't that smell great?" even though smoking has deadened your senses and you can't smell a thing.

No more waking up in the morning and vowing, "*This* is the day I quit."

No more feeling panicky when your only pack is almost empty.

No more wasting money on quit-smoking gimmicks that don't work.

No more oversalting food just so it has some taste.

No more pretending you don't want to quit.

No more feeling smoker's guilt every time your chest hurts.

No more putting off seeing a doctor
because you don't want to discuss your
smoking.

No more ignoring an early warning sign
of cancer because you're afraid the doctor will tell you to quit.

No more lying to yourself that the last
carton you bought really was the last one.

No more sitting on the sidelines because
you don't have the stamina to stay in the
game.

No more telling people you're too old
to quit.

No more fearing that it may be too late to quit.

No more danger of your young child picking up your lighter and mistaking it for a toy.

You told your new boss that you don't smoke.

Your child has started quoting smoking-related health risks.

Your family has a history of heart disease.

You were the only smoker at family gatherings.

You wish you had quit ten years ago.
But ten years from now, you'll be glad
you quit.

You want your future to look bright and
rosy, not dull and ash gray.

You know any tobacco lawsuit settle-
ments are going to come out of smokers'
pockets.

You have better things to do on your
coffee breaks.

You saw a photograph of a guy smoking
through his tracheotomy hole.

You don't want tobacco to win.

Tar keeps rain from leaking through roofs and oxygen from getting through lung walls.

There's a higher resale value for non-smokers' cars.

Radiation treatments.

Chemotherapy.

Hair loss from radiation treatments and chemo.

Hospital gowns don't close in the back.

Hospital food.

Bedpans.

Hospital ventilators.

ICUs are nonsmoking.

Smoking could lead to sky-high doctor bills.

You just had your teeth cleaned and polished.

Smoking makes you ashamed of yourself.

You're tired of this crutch.

You'll endure flu season better.

No more shortness of breath.

There's a big difference between discom-
fort and pain.

Your family is praying for your success.

You're the only team parent who smokes.

You're paying a small fortune in monthly
health-club dues.

You want the sparks in your bedroom to
be from red-hot romance, not from red-
hot cigarettes.

It will be easier to find a date.

You want to gossip at the water cooler, not be banished to the backdoor.

You feel bad that nonsmokers are subjected to your secondhand smoke.

Your folks won't let you smoke in their house.

Your kids won't let you smoke in their houses.

Your friends won't let you smoke in their houses.

Your family won't let you smoke in *your* house.

Once you've kicked the habit, you'll fall asleep faster.

You've got better things to do with your life.

You know what nicotine does to a body.

For yourself, if not for anyone else.

A cigarette never solved a problem.

You're a puff away from a pack a day.

Cancer of the lip.

Cancer of the gum.

Cancer of the palate.

The tobacco industry makes a yearly profit of $13 billion from cigarette sales in the United States.

More than fifty thousand scientific studies have documented a direct link between smoking and disease.

The Surgeon General commented that "smoking represents the most extensively documented cause of disease ever investigated in the history of biomedical research."

The Surgeon General reports cigarette smoking is a contributing cause of brain hemorrhages.

The United States Public Health Service reports have called cigarette smoking the most preventable cause of death in our society.

More than one out of six deaths in the United States are caused by smoking— three times the number killed by cocaine, heroin, and alcohol combined.

The Surgeon General reports cigarette smoking is a contributing cause of aneurysm of the abdominal aorta.

Abnormal Pap smear tests.

Leukemia.

Blood clots in your legs.

You want to look forward to the Great American Smokeout.

World No Tobacco Day is gaining popularity.

That feeling of frustration will pass.

Chronic obstructive pulmonary disease.

Smokers face twice the risk of dying of heart attacks than do nonsmokers.

You bought the gum.

Your quit-date has arrived.

You like the sound of "I don't smoke."

You want to give this attempt to quit
your best shot.

You're as prepared to quit as you'll
ever be.

You can make it through this rough spot.

You know "it's my only vice" is a stupid
rationalization.

Tomorrow never comes; quitting has to
happen today.

You know everyone has to die of something. You just don't want to give that
something a hand.

You made it through the last acute urge.

"Just one more cigarette" is just one more lie.

That intriguing woman in your quit-smoking class.

That interesting gentleman in your quit-smoking group.

There is no safe way to smoke. None.

Smoking causes cancer. Period.

Nicotine is a poison that, if taken in large doses, could kill a person by paralyzing breathing muscles.

You know smoking is unhealthy even if you don't inhale.

Statistically, smokers die ten to twelve years younger than nonsmokers.

You started because you were curious. Now you know.

The tobacco industry spends roughly $6 billion annually to develop and market ads that show smoking as an exciting, glamorous, healthy adult activity.

There are exciting, glamorous, healthy adult activities that don't kill you.

Researchers say that—like alcohol, heroin, and cocaine—nicotine can have a permanent tolerance in the body. When an ex-smoker smokes a cigarette, even years after quitting, the nicotine could quickly hook him or her on the old habit.

The percentage of adults who smoke dropped from 42 percent in 1965 to 25 percent in 1995.

After waking, a smoker coughs because the lungs are trying to expel the poisons built up from the previous day of smoking.

Smokers' lungs are more susceptible to bacteria and viruses than nonsmokers'.

Since 1966, the Surgeon General's health warnings have been required on all cigarette packages and, since 1987, on all containers of smokeless tobacco products.

The United States Congress banned cigarette ads on TV and radio in 1971 and banned ads of smokeless tobacco products in 1987.

The United States health care costs caused directly by smoking total more than $50 billion annually.

Smoking costs the United States more than $50 billion each year in lost economic productivity.

More than forty million Americans have successfully quit smoking.

Colorectal cancer.

Colostomies.

Photographs of smokers' lungs.

Those wrinkles around your mouth.

With regard to quitting, you've come a long way, baby.

Smoking reduces fertility.

Smoking is *not* a simple pleasure.

When it comes to smoking, if you keep your head buried in the sand, the rest of you will join it all too soon.

No more waking up afraid that you didn't snub out that late-night cigarette.

No more rushing phone conversations because you couldn't reach your smokes.

As James Brown might say, you want to feel good—*NAH nah NAH nah NAH nah NAH*—the way that you should, yeah!

You want to simplify your life.

You want to know how clean mountain air *really* smells.

Your recreational vehicle has become a Li'l Smoker on wheels.

You used to run marathons.

Each time you light up, you feel like a schnook.

You suspect when you push away the ashtray as soon as you've snubbed out a cigarette, your subconscious is trying to tell you something.

You don't want to disappoint a lot of people, especially yourself.

You're tired of people laughing when you say you're concerned about air pollution.

This can be the first day of the rest of
your smoke-free life.

No more fidgeting through long religious
services.

Deep down, you suspect smoking may be
a sin.

Nonsmokers are getting the promotions
at work.

Nonsmoking company cars.

Someday you want to walk your daughter
down the aisle.

Someday you want to spoil your grandkids.

You want to see the day when your teens have teens.

You want to be a grandma like your grandma was.

You want to shut up the people who chirp, "If I can quit, you can, too!"

Friends won't let you smoke in their cars.

You're not allowed to smoke in malls.

The price you pay for smoking is a lot more than the cost of cigarettes.

No more looking like a cheapskate when you bum smokes.

You're tired of flipping over the pack so you can't see the Surgeon General's health warning.

More room in those little purses.

You'd like to actually taste those fancy restaurant meals you've been buying.

Let's face it: Smoking is a disgusting habit.

At the end of a day of heavy smoking, you feel rotten.

Precancerous cells.

People you've met recently act disappointed when they learn you smoke.

Your best friend will quit if you do.

Exploratory surgery.

You only started on a dare.

Today is an excellent day to quit.

You're looking forward to the day when you're not obsessed with smoking . . . and not obsessed with not smoking.

No more really nasty-looking spit.

You have a "life wish."

You quit, remember?

Your cat won't stink of smoke.

No more ashes in the—oh shoot!—
pots and pans while cooking.

Your child's incredibly long school
pageant.

Long ballets.

Very long operas.

Your favorite doctor—the one who
smoked—died at age sixty of lung cancer.

Five extra pounds is much less of a
health risk than continuing to smoke.

It's just a habit.

You know a troop leader shouldn't be
lighting up on overnight campouts.

Polyps.

Temporarily out-of-service elevators.

Hiking.

Backpacking.

Jogging.

In-line skating.

Your teenager has challenged you to a racquetball game.

You were the only one in the neighborhood still smoking.

Perfume doesn't cover the smell of smoke.

You'd like to die peacefully in your sleep—a long time from now.

You don't like being hooked on anything.

More money for car toys.

It's a new year!

Your girlfriend gave you an ultimatum.

Your boyfriend said he's tired of "kissing an ashtray."

No more stinky telephone.

You're creating a whole new you, inside and out.

Fish can smell smoke on your lures and flies.

You've noticed your child's teddy bear stinks of smoke.

You're not interested in committing suicide—quickly or slowly.

You want your life to be better than it has been.

Your nieces and nephews admire you.

Smoking only socially is like being only a little bit pregnant.

Tobacco companies don't have "trade in your empty pack for a new pack" booths at car racetracks because their executives are swell guys.

You already have enough health problems. You don't need any more.

You just painted the inside of your house.

No one really wants smoke in his or her lungs.

You want your mourners to say, "At least he had a long, long life."

When you cut the grass, you're wheezing more than your old gas lawnmower.

You said you'd quit when you finished high school.

You said you'd quit when you left for college.

You said you'd quit when you graduated from college.

You said you'd quit when you got married.

You said you'd quit before the baby was born.

You said you'd quit before the kids were old enough to realize what you were doing.

You said you'd quit before your kids became teens.

You said you'd quit before your kids grew up and had kids.

You said you'd quit before you retired.

You said you'd quit when you retired.

You said you'd quit before it was too late.

You said you'd quit.

Your pearly white smile used to be your most attractive feature.

You like dozing in front of the TV without the risk of having a dropped lit cigarette burn down the house.

You're horrified that a new generation is taking up the habit.

You're horrified that a new generation is taking up the habit even earlier than yours did.

You're horrified that when you buy cigarettes, you help tobacco companies promote smoking to that new generation.

You haven't been smoking for a very long time.

You *have* been smoking for a very long time.

Smoking doesn't make you look like a 1930s movie star.

Smoking doesn't make you look like a 1940s movie star.

Smoking doesn't make you look like a 1950s movie star.

Smoking doesn't make you look like a 1960s movie star.

Smoking doesn't make you look like a 1970s movie star.

Smoking doesn't make you look like a 1980s movie star.

Smoking doesn't make you look like a 1990s movie star.

Smoking doesn't make you look like a twenty-first century movie star.

You want to collect every penny that was put into your pension fund.

Humans are built to run on oxygen, not smoke.

EKGs.

After you quit, no one can ever call you a wimp.

Smoking does a lot more *to* you than *for* you.

Your guardian angel can see you a lot better without smoke in her eyes.

Your next cigarette could easily lead to the one after that.

Your next cigarette could easily lead to the one after the one after that.

Your next cigarette could easily lead to
the next pack.

Your next cigarette could easily lead to
the next carton.

Your next cigarette could easily lead to
the next $100 spent on smokes.

Your next cigarette could easily lead to
the next $1,000 spent on smokes.

Your next cigarette could easily lead to
another day of smoking.

Your next cigarette could easily lead to
another week of smoking.

Your next cigarette could easily lead to
another month of smoking.

Your next cigarette could easily lead to
another year of smoking.

Your next cigarette could easily lead to
another decade of smoking.

Your next cigarette could easily lead to
exactly where you don't want to be.

Boot-hill.

Buying the farm.

Pushing up daisies.

Taking the big dirt nap.

You want to be around to see your daughter get her degree.

You want to be around to tease your son about his bald spot.

You want to be around to be the matriarch of the family.

You want to be around to be the patriarch of the family.

You want to be around to teach your granddaughter how to sew.

You want to be around to teach your grandson how to throw a curve ball.

You want to be around to brag about your grandkids.

You want to be around to see what electronic marvels come next.

You want to be around when the mortgage is finally paid off.

You want to be around to see the fads and fashions of your youth be in style again

You're looking forward to traveling after you retire.

You're looking forward to smashing your alarm clock after you retire.

You're looking forward to having retirement years outnumber work years.

You're looking forward to getting in shape.

You're looking forward to the day when climbing a hill isn't daunting.

You're looking forward to lasting all morning without coughing.

You're looking forward to lots of pats on the back from friends who are ex-smokers.

You're looking forward to asking out that certain someone who doesn't date smokers.

You're looking forward to your spouse realizing that this time you really have quit.

Quitting for good is quitting for your good.

It'll be so great to brag about quitting.

Because you aren't going to miss seeing the price of a carton pop up on the cash register.

Because you aren't going to miss the disappointed looks on your kids' faces when you light up.

Because you aren't going to miss hoping clients won't smell smoke on your breath.

Because you aren't going to miss defending your smoking.

Because you aren't going to miss cringing at antismoking public-service announcements.

Because you aren't going to miss making nicotine come first.

Because you aren't going to miss thinking about what smoking is doing to you.

Because you aren't going to miss purses littered with tobacco crumbs.

Because you aren't going to miss feeling disappointed when you light up after vowing to quit.

Because you aren't going to miss all those broken promises about quitting.

Because you aren't going to miss trying desperately to scrape one last light from a lighter that's out of fluid.

Because you don't want to miss out on the last part of your life.

Because you don't want to miss out on your granddaughter's First Communion.

Because you don't want to miss out on your grandson's bar mitzvah.

Because you don't want to miss out on telling your grandchildren what their father was like when he was their age.

Because you don't want to miss out on senior discounts.

Because you don't want to miss out on the last 50 percent of your life.

Because you don't want to miss out on the last 40 percent of your life.

Because you don't want to miss out on the last 30 percent of your life.

Because you don't want to miss out on the last 20 percent of your life.

Because you don't want to miss out on the last 10 percent of your life.

Because you don't want to miss out on the last 5 percent of your life.

Because you don't want to miss out on even the last 1 percent of your life.

Because life is risky enough without smoking.

You can't remember why you started.

You never in your wildest dreams imagined you'd still be smoking at this age.

Quitting is a gift for the whole family.

You won't get to baby-sit the grandkids
if you smoke.

It gets lonely smoking on the patio . . . all
by yourself . . . in the middle of winter.

Your dad never quit.

You don't think God is ready for you yet,
and you're sure you're not ready to meet
Him.

This is your chance to start over.

Co-ed softball.

Cross-country skiing.

Sometimes you can't catch your breath.

CAT scans.

You used to be an athlete.

No more feet that are all pins and needles.

You don't want to be a drug addict.

The only thing you want to be addicted
to is love.

Smoking ain't worth being that slim,
Virginia.

You don't even like those young movie
stars who smoke.

You don't want your money to go up in smoke.

You don't want your health to go up in smoke.

You don't want that special relationship to go up in smoke.

You don't want your future to go up in smoke.

You don't want your promotion to go up in smoke.

You don't want your love life to go up in smoke.

You don't want your newfound self-esteem to go up in smoke.

You don't want your parents' pride that you quit to go up in smoke.

You don't want your kids' congratulations on your quitting to go up in smoke.

You don't want your recovery from surgery to go up in smoke.

You don't want your hard-fought victory over addiction to go up in smoke.

You don't want your life to go up in smoke.

You used to be the jump rope champ.

Bowling leaves you breathless.

You lose your breath just bending over to tie your shoes.

Nonsmoking friends have been able to smell you coming.

Life is already too short.

Lungs were meant to last a lifetime.

The wizard may not be able to find you a new heart.

Respiratory therapists.

You have a bigger craving to live a long life.

Your daughter is pregnant.

Your granddaughter is pregnant.

You've told your friends and family your quit-date.

Your next puff will lead to a lot of huffing and puffing.

More wind to yell at stupid drivers.

The pleasure of one more cigarette isn't worth the pain of going through all this again.

You'll have the perfect excuse for being a little portly . . . for a while, anyway.

It's time to exercise, not to smoke.

The American Heart Association.

The American Cancer Society.

The American Lung Association.

A recent relapse isn't a reason to give up.

Researchers say secondhand smoke is the third leading cause of preventable death in the United States.

Secondhand smoke kills fifty-three thousand nonsmokers in the United States every year.

Secondhand smoke kills more than 4,400 nonsmokers in the United States every month.

Secondhand smoke kills more than one thousand nonsmokers in the United States every week.

Secondhand smoke kills 145 nonsmokers in the United States every day.

Secondhand smoke kills six nonsmokers in the United States every hour.

Secondhand smoke kills one nonsmoker in the United States every ten minutes.

Secondhand smoke kills nonsmokers who begged their loved ones to quit smoking.

Worldwide, three million people die every year as a result of smoking.

Worldwide, 250,000 people die every month as a result of smoking.

Worldwide, over fifty-seven thousand people die every week as a result of smoking.

Worldwide, over eight thousand people die every day as a result of smoking.

Worldwide, over three hundred people
die every hour as a result of smoking.

Worldwide, five people die every minute
as a result of smoking.

Worldwide, one person dies every twelve
seconds as a result of smoking.

You've drawn a line in the sand—
or in the ash, anyway.

Defibrillators.

IVs.

Rib spreaders.

Physical therapy.

Occupational therapy.

You're out of sick leave.

You don't want tobacco to win.

You want to improve your golf game.

Your rabbi.

Your priest.

Your minister.

Your pastor.

Your shaman.

Smoking is against your religion.

The Bible.

The Torah.

The Koran.

The commandment that says, "Thou shalt not kill."

Your bouncing baby boy.

Your darling little girl.

Your infant keeps staring at you.

Your toddler pointed at your cigarette pack and asked, "What's that?"

Your preschooler pretended his straw was a cigarette.

Your grade-schooler did a report on smoking and health.

Your junior high student has friends who smoke.

Your high schooler said she'll quit when you do.

Your college student doesn't need another reason to think you're not too bright.

Your twenty-something child still needs your advice.

Your middle-aged child still believes this time you'll succeed.

A spring breeze that smells of honey-suckle.

Brisk jaunts through the woods.

The crystal clear air of a winter morning.

You don't want to buy a new pack.

You don't want to bum another cigarette.

You hate being politically incorrect.

Eventually, your body will really like being nicotine-free.

You want to play your saxophone, trumpet, or tuba again.

Scuba gear works better with lungs that work well.

You've promised yourself a trip to an island paradise if you quit.

You want to smile in photographs without showing smoker's teeth.

You've overheard your friends complain that after being around you, their hair and clothes stink of smoke.

Nervousness is better than nerve damage.

Cancer wards.

You would rather not develop a devotion to St. Peregrine, the patron saint of cancer patients.

You just spent a bundle on a complete-gym machine.

This is what separates the men from the boys and the women from the girls.

It's hard to look chic when you're hacking up phlegm.

Stain-free fingernails.

Women are supposed to be smarter than men. Your husband quit.

Men are supposed to be stronger than women. Your wife quit.

No more worrying about what blind dates will think about your habit.

Your dad's going to give you a pat on the back when you succeed.

Being in shape requires being smoke-free.

You're tired of being a "closet smoker."

Cough, cough, *COUGH*, cough, cough.

That famous daredevil doesn't smoke because he considers it too risky.

Ashes on the floor of your car.

Ashes on your car door outside your "flicking" window.

People with good taste—literally, a good sense of taste—don't smoke.

You're tired of having a butt dangling between your lips.

You never could figure out how to keep a pack rolled up in your T-shirt sleeve.

Cutting back didn't work.

You no longer want to huddle with the smokers at the side door of the office building, yearning to breath freely.

You want to be done with this and get on with the rest of your life.

You don't want to die before your parents do.

Your parents don't want you to die before they do.

Quitting sets a good example for your younger brothers and sisters.

Setting up strict guidelines about where and when you'll smoke didn't work.

Quitting cold turkey is better than ending up a dead duck.

Smoking makes you feel like a chump.

Smoking, by definition, sucks.

You feel sick when you think of all the money you've already wasted on smokes.

When you consider the price of a cigarette pack, quitting is like getting free money.

Years ago, you vowed to never spend more than a nickel a pack.

Years ago, you vowed to never spend more than a dime a pack.

Years ago, you vowed to never spend
more than a quarter a pack.

Years ago, you vowed to never spend
more than a half-dollar a pack.

Years ago, you vowed to never spend
more than six bits a pack.

Years ago, you vowed to never spend
more than a dollar a pack.

Years ago, you vowed to never spend
more than a buck and a half a pack.

Years ago, you vowed to never spend
more than two bucks a pack.

Years ago, you vowed to never spend
more than two and a half dollars a pack.

There's no way around the hard part of
quitting.

No more stifled sneezes that produce
little puffs of smoke.

You no longer want to live in a self-made
gas chamber.

You're tired of living under a cloud.

Lungs are designed to go *out* with the
bad and *in* with the good.

Your dog inhales your secondhand smoke.

Your nonsmoking coworkers will be so proud you quit that they'll buy you lunch in the cafe's nonsmoking section.

Your nonsmoking friends will be so proud you quit that they'll buy you dinner in the restaurant's nonsmoking section.

Your nonsmoking spouse will be so proud you quit that the two of you will have a smokin' evening now that you're not smoking.

Your ex-smoking friends are going to be so happy for you.

Your smoking friends are going to be so jealous of you.

The side effects of withdrawal prove
what a powerful drug nicotine is.

Nobody ever died of carrot sticks.

That dizzy spell you didn't tell anyone
about.

Sometimes it hurts when you take a deep
breath.

You want a little more Zip-A-Dee in your
Doo-Dah.

Climbing the walls can be considered
aerobic exercise.

Tumors.

You don't want your unofficial epitaph to be "She finally quit."

Hell is depicted as fire, brimstone . . . and smoke.

You want your home to be your castle, not a smokehouse.

You want to be able to enjoy parties at the homes of nonsmoking friends.

You want nonsmoking friends to enjoy parties at your home.

You want not just quantity but quality of life.

Tomorrow morning is going to be terrific
if you don't light up tonight.

Quit-smoking scare tactics are so frightening because they're true.

The journey of thousands of smokeless
days begins with one day of not smoking.

You can't deny you've been living in
denial.

You claim to be an environmentalist.

You say you want what's best for your
children.

Your kid's allergies.

You don't want your children going to school stinking of smoke.

There's a reason they're called *coffin nails*.

You're tired of walking into the store and thinking, "I shouldn't buy these. I shouldn't buy these. I shouldn't buy these."

You want to take up tae kwon do.

You can't remember the last time you heard someone list the benefits of smoking.

Smoking and yoga don't mix.

Sometimes you feel like you're drowning, and quitting is your only lifeline.

You cringe when you think of how many cigarettes you've already smoked.

If God had wanted you to smoke, He would have made you with a chimney, not a respiratory system.

Nonsmoking rental cars.

You promised your fiancé.

You promised your fiancée.

No more dirty looks from your in-laws.

The only way to make your smoking
ancient history is to not light up here
and now.

You are now in the nonsmoking section
of your life. And you want to stay there.

Smoking didn't make you more witty.

Smoking didn't make you more hand-
some.

Smoking didn't make you prettier.

Smoking didn't make you more alluring.

Smoking didn't help you win friends and
influence people.

Smoking didn't make you smarter.

Smoking didn't make you stronger.

Smoking didn't make you more athletic.

Smoking didn't fill your life with grace and blessings.

Smoking didn't make you a better person.

Smoking didn't do anything for you but make you a smoker . . . and put your health at risk . . . and cost you a lot of money.

Money spent on cigarettes can now go to charity.

Money spent on cigarettes can now go toward your boat fund.

Money spent on cigarettes can now go toward purchasing premium cable.

Money spent on cigarettes can now go toward buying new clothes.

Money spent on cigarettes can now go toward getting top-of-the-line running shoes.

Money spent on cigarettes can now go toward renewing a health club membership.

Money spent on cigarettes can now go toward leasing a better apartment.

Money spent on cigarettes can now go
toward paying off the mortgage faster.

Money spent on cigarettes can now go
toward buying dinners at places where
they don't ask, "You want fries with that?"

Money spent on cigarettes can now go
toward paying for weekends at bed-and-
breakfasts.

Quitting has been on your to-do list long
enough.

Smoking was the old you.

You're one old dog who's ready to learn
a new trick.

You still wish your mother had quit
before she got sick and died.

Your kids need you even if they are
middle-aged. (What do *they* know?)

It's time to heal.

The pain will be temporary; the pride
will last the rest of your lifetime.

You've survived tougher times than these.

Quitting is worth the effort.

You believe the quit-smoking literature
and statistics.

Deep down, you think not quitting is even more frightening than quitting.

"Forever" is nothing but a lot of "right nows."

You no longer need to smoke to prove you're grown up.

Quitting was your birthday wish.

Quitting is a giant step in the right direction.

Your grandchildren have been parroting antismoking TV ads.

Suicide by degrees is still suicide.

Your teenaged grandchild has argued, "But Grandpa smokes."

Tobacco companies may still argue for an appeal, but the verdict is in: Smoking is an addiction that can kill.

What started out as a lark has turned into an albatross.

You had no intention of smoking a year.

You had no intention of smoking two years.

You had no intention of smoking three years.

You had no intention of smoking four
years.

You had no intention of smoking five
years.

You had no intention of smoking ten
years.

You had no intention of smoking fifteen
years.

You had no intention of smoking twenty
years.

You had no intention of smoking twenty-
five years.

You had no intention of smoking thirty years.

You had no intention of smoking thirty-five years.

You had no intention of smoking forty years.

You had no intention of smoking forty-five years.

You had no intention of smoking fifty years.

You had no intention of smoking the rest of your life.

You always assumed you'd be an ex-smoker at this point in your life.

Two-hour classes without breaks.

Long bus rides with few rest stops.

You can make this the first day of your better life.

More razzle in your dazzle.

More energy to play on the weekends.

Willpower is like a muscle: It gets stronger each time you flex it.

You'll be able to charge right up the stairs
if the elevator is too slow in coming.

No more getting winded just walking
across the parking lot.

You want to try race walking.

You want to try skydiving. Once.

You want to try handball.

You want to try tap-dancing.

You want to try rock climbing.

You want to try hang-gliding.

You want to try running around the track at the high school.

You want to try kayaking.

You want to try mountain climbing.

You want to try walking two miles a day.

You want to try rec-league soccer.

You want to try whatever sport you feel like trying.

You can't remember the last time you felt just fine first thing in the morning.

You can't remember the last time you felt this proud about something you have done.

You can't remember the last time you did something really great by yourself for yourself.

You can't remember the last time you wanted to be something as badly as you want to be an ex-smoker.

You can't remember the last time you didn't feel guilty buying smokes.

You can't remember the last time you were glad you smoked.

You can't remember the last time you felt really great.

You can't remember the last time you were pleased someone cool found out you smoked.

You can't remember the last time you argued that smoking was a really good idea.

You can't remember the last time you sat through a staff meeting without desperately craving your next cigarette.

You can't remember the last time you didn't think twice about an upcoming physical exam.

Tomorrow you're going to tell your quit-smoking group you made it through today smoke-free.

Tomorrow you're going to tell your spouse you made it through today smoke-free.

Tomorrow you're going to tell your kids you made it through today smoke-free.

Tomorrow you're going to tell your ex-smoking coworkers you made it through today smoke-free.

Tomorrow you're going to tell your cyberspace friends you made it through today smoke-free.

Tomorrow you're going to tell your neighbors you made it through today smoke-free.

Tomorrow you're going to tell your boss you made it through today smoke-free.

Tomorrow you're going to tell your staff you made it through today smoke-free.

Tomorrow you're going to tell your grandkids you made it through today smoke-free.

Tomorrow you're going to tell your parents you made it through today smoke-free.

Tomorrow you're going to tell your grandparents you made it through today smoke-free.

Tomorrow you're going to tell your siblings you made it through today smoke-free.

Tomorrow you're going to tell the world you made it through today smoke-free.

Investigators determined the cause of the fire was a cigarette.

Singed mustache hairs.

MRIs.

Grim-faced doctors.

This may be your last chance.

Anything this hard to do must have a *big* payoff.

You're old but would like to get older.

You no longer need to smoke to stay alert in some foxhole.

You know you have to stop.

Any smoking is too much smoking.

Smoking socially is like inhaling poisonous gases in a pleasant setting.

The hell of quitting is the only way to the heaven of being an ex-smoker.

The importance of quitting really is as serious as a heart attack.

The best way to light up someone's life is not to light up.

Health insurance deductibles.

Health insurance copayments.

The cost of prescriptions.

Lab tests that come back positive for abnormalities.

Peer pressure to quit.

Four-floor walkups.

No other animal inhales smoke on purpose.

You feel trapped, but you know quitting is the only way out.

You've put a lot of money into your retirement account.

The "smoking" room at work is an old broom closet.

Making it through today will give you a running start on tomorrow.

Catheters.

Addiction isn't glamorous.

You don't have to be a genius to know
you should quit, but you'll be a moron if
you don't.

It's a childish habit that you began when
you were a child.

You're not sure what an oral fixation is,
but you're pretty sure you don't want one.

Each little success leads to a complete
victory.

You can inhale all the fumes you want
for free by keeping your car window
down on the freeway.

Smoking is a wretched habit.

It's a vile habit.

It's the habit you hate the most.

No matter how hard you've tried, you can't forget what the doctor said.

That first heart attack might have been your last warning.

Being jittery is better than being comatose.

You want a life that isn't nicotine-centric.

If tobacco companies really want to give appropriate gifts, they should offer smokers coupons for tombstones.

There's a reason your children have been hiding your smokes.

For a long time, you've felt chained to your cigarettes.

No one ever thought your IQ was higher because you had a butt dangling between your lips.

No amount or variety of vitamins can compensate for the effects of smoking.

Clean lungs.

Clear arteries.

A brain that isn't pickling in the chemicals found in cigarette smoke.

Looking forward to the day when you don't miss cigarettes.

Looking forward to the time in your life when all this is just an unpleasant memory.

The joy of walking right by the smokers standing around outside your office building.

The look on the face of that smoking coworker who considers you a weenie.

You have the power to make your loved ones' greatest wish come true.

You want to grow old and wear purple.

Reaching a birthday you wouldn't have seen if you'd kept smoking.

Nicotine withdrawal won't kill you. Smoking will.

Withdrawal is the ransom you pay for letting nicotine kidnap your body.

Increased libido. (Wink, wink.)

You don't want strangers reading your obituary to say, "Too bad. She was so young."

You've got a lot of living to do.

There's no better Christmas gift for your family.

The Grim Reaper carries a lighter.

Millions of dead smokers thought medical science would come up with a magical cure just in time.

Addiction can be overcome one miserable moment at a time.

The sun can come up tomorrow on an ex-smoking you.

Looking in the mirror and shouting, "I did it! I did it! I did it!"

Your body will thank you.

You don't want to spend your senior years kicking yourself in the rear for not quitting now.

You know too much now to ever really enjoy smoking again.

You've become accustomed to breathing.

Children yet to be born.

Grandchildren yet to be imagined.

Quitting tells family and friends "I love you."

The problem with not quitting is you can't blame anyone else for your mistake.

Going through withdrawal is part of the high cost of living.

You are a rational being.

The human body and cigarette smoke don't mix.

You want your life's story to have a happy ending.

Forcing a prisoner to smoke would be considered cruel and unusual punishment.

Stairs have gotten steeper.

You want to do what your heart is telling you to do.

There's no point in waiting. Science is never going to come up with a magic pill that makes quitting easy.

It took you more than a few days to get hooked; it will take more than a few days to get unhooked.

There are worse things than quitting, which is why you want to quit.

The first definition of nicotine is "a poisonous alkaloid."

You can't reverse the aging process, but quitting will slam on the brakes.

You don't want your hopes, plans, and goals to be only pipe dreams.

No one ever died too early from quitting too soon.

You've dropped all those other stupid habits you picked up as a teen.

You're tired of being angry at yourself about smoking.

Your lungs never did anything to hurt you.

Just about every illness, disease, or affliction is compounded by smoking.

This will be a big change with big rewards.

Your true friends want you to succeed.

You know each cigarette is taking time off your life.

The only way to quit is to quit.

Saying *no* to your next cigarette is saying *yes* to thousands of good things.

Folks who say quitting was hard but worth it aren't just blowing smoke.

You're tired of nicotine telling you what to do.

Your conscience has been screaming for a long time now.

Ignoring what smoking does to you won't stop smoking from doing those things to you.

Your "closet smoking" isn't fooling anyone.

After you succeed, you'll feel reborn.

You love yourself.

Everyone knows one person who smoked until she was in her eighties—and dozens of smokers who died in their sixties.

Your coworkers are tired of covering your extra smoke-breaks.

Quitting is a death-defying act.

You want a little more pep in the romance department.

You've seen the look on your wife's face when you light up.

Your husband is scared for you and for him and for the kids.

A stress reliever that adds stress to your life isn't helpful.

Lately, your lungs have been congested until midmorning.

You want to make it beyond the warm-ups on the step-aerobics videotape.

You want to report success at your next Nicotine Anonymous meeting.

The amount spent on ten cartons could buy a really big TV set.

You won't just live longer, you'll live better.

You don't want friends and family to sit around someday discussing the size of your tumor.

You're tired of wheezing like a broken bagpipe.

The only remorse you'll feel after quitting is not quitting sooner.

Your mama told you not to smoke.

Lately, that little pack has felt like a ball and chain.

You'll get all the credit for quitting. And you will have earned it.

Quitting is a matter of when and how, not if.

You're not just older, you're wiser.

Life is precious.

Quitting is like taking a long, cool drink from the fountain of youth.

It's been years since your friends thought smoking was cool.

No one feels as alive as a new ex-smoker.

The little voice inside your head is speaking the truth.

A smoky future never looks bright.

Not smoking is a virtue that offers more than its own reward.

No tobacco company offers enough bonus coupons for a lung transplant.

Tobacco companies know why their markets have to be replenished constantly.

Now that you've reached thirty, it's starting to dawn on you that someday you'll be forty.

Now that you've reached forty, you realize forty isn't so old.

Now that you've reached sixty, you want to stick around to collect your social security.

There's no other way except quitting. (If there were, someone would have figured it out a long time ago.)

A smoker is never really free.

One x-ray is worth a thousand words.

Kicking the habit will add bounce to your step.

Pretty soon, being smoke-free will feel as natural as breathing.

You want to enjoy your senior years.

Cigarettes don't taste as good as they used to.

Your half-quitting measures have proven to be half-baked.

You don't have to be crazy to start smoking, but it's crazy not to quit.

You want to start dating again.

The benefits of smoking don't outweigh its risks.

You're tired of breathing heavily when you climb a flight of stairs.

You used to enjoy dancing.

Wheezing doesn't sound sexy.

Only you can make this dream come true.

If you're smoking OPs—other people's cigarettes—you're still smoking.

Blowing smoke rings has lost its charm.

It's a lot better to have clean lungs and chewed-up fingernails than filthy lungs and stained fingernails.

Quitting is the gift your family really wants from you.

How many times have you promised to quit?

You don't want to be the last one in your group to quit smoking—or the first to lose a lung.

You want to put NS (nonsmoker) in your next personal ad.

You can get cancer in places you didn't even know you had.

Angioplasty may be a relatively safe procedure, but it's a lot safer to quit smoking.

Your parents still blame themselves for not stopping you when you first started smoking.

Throat lozenges can't cure what ails you.

Your grandchild wants to hear stories about when you were a kid.

Smoking might seem like a really good idea to a fifteen-year-old, but you're not fifteen anymore.

The tide of public opinion has turned: Smoking isn't cool anymore.

New upholstered furniture.

Your loved ones would do it for you if they could.

Your success will encourage your smoking friends to quit.

Now that you've reached fifty, you're looking forward to getting your senior discount.

Now that you've reached seventy, odds are you won't see eighty if you don't quit.

Quitting isn't the problem. It's the solution.

No more burn marks on your countertops.

Better to lose a habit than to lose a lung.

It's been too long since you could jog three miles.

You would rather not keep funding the tobacco industries' $500-per-hour lawyers.

The Surgeon General wasn't kidding when he wrote those warnings.

The harder it is to quit, the better you'll feel when you do it.

Many cigarette-ad cowboys have died of lung cancer.

The money you'll save from smoking a pack a day will buy you a $1,000 gift in just one year.

It's getting too hard trying not to think about the consequences of smoking.

The family has gone to enough funerals in recent years.

It's a new day.

It's a new month.

It's a new year.

It's a new century.

It's a new millennium.

No ex-smoker has ever said, "Gee, I wish I had kept the habit just a *little* longer."

You don't stick forks in toasters, so why suck cigarette smoke into your lungs?

Smoking a cigarette occasionally is as smart as occasionally hitting yourself on the head with a hammer.

The advertising image of the energetic, sophisticated smoker is just a smoke screen.

Your kids want you to quit as much as you want them never to start.

Cigarette smoke may be gray, but the facts of smoking are black and white.

It's hard to grab the brass ring with a cigarette in your hand.

The road to recovery is uphill, but it's well worth the climb.

No one else can quit for you; quitting is up to you.

You're tired of making a cigarette the axis around which your world turns.

You don't want your spouse to become your caregiver.

You can't brush your lungs clean like you can your teeth.

You're exhausted.

Your chest hurts in one particular spot.

There are no safe brands of smokes.

When you retire, you'll know each day is a blessing. And cutting that time short by even one day would be a tragedy.

The key to your willpower is your "won't power."

The lining of a cloud of cigarette smoke is anything but silver.

Nicotine is the hook; tobacco advertising is the line; cancer is the sinker.

House paid off. Kids grown up. Retirement income set. Why let smoking steal what might be the best decades of your life?

Putting your hands over your ears and singing *la la la la* won't change the truth.

You deserve better health.

Each cigarette sucks the life out of you.

Unlike hell, heaven is nonsmoking.

Chain-smoking has shackled your life.

Those little "boosts" you get when you smoke aren't worth the crashing and burning that comes later.

You don't want your midtwenties to end up being your middle-aged years.

You want to be around to hold your great-grandchild.

You've already put enough tar through your system to fill a good-sized pothole.

Everyone needs good lungs because most of life is uphill.

Someday you'll want to have eighty candles on your birthday cake.

Smoking is counterproductive.

You haven't written your memoirs yet.

You haven't danced at your daughter's wedding yet.

You haven't spoiled your grandchildren yet.

You haven't enjoyed your first day of retirement yet.

You haven't taken that cruise yet.

You and your spouse haven't smooched in a European capital yet.

You haven't learned to play the piano yet.

You haven't checked off half the things on your lifetime to-do list.

No more dreading when friends say, "It's only a couple of blocks. Let's walk."

No more feeling exhausted before you even get to work.

No more measuring time by the number of cigarettes you've smoked that day.

No more steering the conversation away from smoking.

You've prayed about quitting.

You'd like a little more juice in your batteries.

You don't want to smoke, and you're tired of needing to.

You have the power to change.

Quitting can be the cornerstone of the foundation for a new life.

Quitting isn't an easy goal, but it's an attainable one.

The willpower you're developing now will help you in countless other ways later.

The scent of lilacs on a warm spring day.

The surprise inside every cigarette isn't like the one inside a Cracker Jack box.

FYI: Quitting PDQ can help prevent you from being DOA.

You promised your valentine you'd quit.

You don't have money to burn.

You'd like to actually taste that fancy-schmancy coffee you've been drinking lately.

No more smoking hiccups from inhaling too fast.

Your only old once, if you're lucky.

You've decided you actually *would* like
to live forever.

You can think of even *more* reasons to quit.